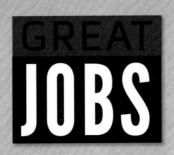

Great Jobs in Health Care

Barbara Sheen

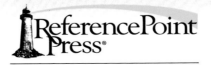

ReferencePoint Press®

San Diego, CA

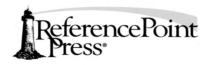

About the Author
Barbara Sheen is the author of 101 books for young people. She lives in New Mexico with her family. In her spare time, she likes to swim, walk, garden, and cook.

For more information, contact:
ReferencePoint Press, Inc.
PO Box 27779
San Diego, CA 92198
www.ReferencePointPress.com

Picture Credits:

Cover: damircudic/iStockphoto.com
 7: Maury Aaseng
13: Antonio Guillem/Shutterstock.com
29: Africa Studio/Shutterstock.com
52: FatCamera/iStockphoto.com
67: iStockphoto.com

LIBRARY OF CONGRESS CATALOGING-IN-PUBLICATION DATA

Name: Sheen, Barbara, author.
Title: Great Jobs in Health Care/by Barbara Sheen.
Description: San Diego, CA: ReferencePoint Press, Inc., 2019. | Series:
  Great Jobs | Audience: Grade 9 to 12. | Includes bibliographical
  references and index.
Identifiers: LCCN 2018034647 (print) | LCCN 2018035334 (ebook) | ISBN
  9781682825242 (eBook) | ISBN 9781682825235 (hardback)
Subjects: LCSH: Medicine—Vocational guidance—Juvenile literature. | Medical
  personnel—Juvenile literature.
Classification: LCC R690 (ebook) | LCC R690 .S473 2019 (print) | DDC
  610.69—dc23
LC record available at https://lccn.loc.gov/2018034647

Contents

Making a Difference

Anyone who enjoys helping others and wants to make a positive difference in the world should consider a career in health care. On a daily basis, the actions of health care professionals change—and often save—lives. "Not a day goes by where I don't have an opportunity . . . to solve somebody's unique problem," blogger and physician assistant Stephen Pasquini explains in an article on the Physician Assistant Life website. "It doesn't have to be a cure for Malaria, just providing a curative treatment plan for your patient's hemorrhoids can have a remarkable effect on a person's life."

A Large Career Field

With more than 10 million workers and over two hundred different careers, the health care industry is one of the nation's largest employers. Many, but not all, health care professionals work directly with patients, providing diverse services to individuals ranging from newborns to the elderly. For example, phlebotomists, sonographers, and nuclear medicine technologists administer medical tests. Optometrists, ophthalmologists, and ophthalmic technicians examine and care for eyes. Psychiatrists, psychologists, mental health counselors, and art and music therapists help people cope with mental and emotional issues. Other health care professionals set broken bones, deliver babies, perform surgery, administer anesthesia, improve the speech and language skills of people with communication disorders, and help disabled people overcome physical limitations. Indeed, the many services these professionals perform could fill a book—or many books.

Some health care professionals do not work directly with patients; but they, too, help others. Through their work, they make it possible for those who work directly with patients to do their jobs. These individuals keep medical facilities running smoothly. Hospital administrators, for instance, are in charge of hospitals and medical centers, where they manage personnel, handle budgets and scheduling, and purchase equipment, among other tasks. Other health care professionals maintain patient records, schedule appointments, and handle medical billing. Some repair medical equipment, while others, such as biomedical engineers, develop new medical technologies; still others, known as medical scientists, search for cures, preventions, and treatments for diseases and medical conditions. Belgian neurologist and medical scientist Steven Laureys is a member of the latter group. He studies brain activity of coma patients. In an interview on the website of the medical engineering firm Guger Technologies, Laureys explains, "It is wonderful to be paid to think, and push the frontiers of our knowledge . . . to be able to see the effects of your research directly translated to diagnostic and prognostic problems."

A Hot Field

With so many possible careers in health care, there is something to suit almost everyone's interests, personality, and skills. Unlike other industries that are losing jobs, the health care industry is growing rapidly. In fact, the Bureau of Labor Statistics projects that health care will be the fastest-growing employment sector through at least 2024. This means that qualified individuals should be able to find suitable employment. Once they are employed, health care professionals can expect to have more job security than individuals in other sectors. And they can choose to work in a variety of settings almost anywhere in the world. They work in hospitals, clinics, nursing homes, and private medical practices. They work in military facilities, schools, research laboratories, and government agencies, among other settings. Some, such as home health aides and visiting nurses, care for patients in the patient's private residence.

Moreover, many health care careers are financially rewarding. Fifteen of the top twenty-five jobs in *U.S. News & World Report*'s annual ranking of the best-paying jobs for 2018 were in health care. Salaries for highly trained professionals like physicians and dentists can reach well into six figures. Many health care professionals receive generous employee benefits that include health insurance, educational reimbursement plans, and paid sick leave and vacations.

Another benefit is flexible hours. Some health care professionals work eight hours per day, five days a week. Many others work part time. Some work in shifts. They may work seven days on, followed by seven days off or work twelve-hour shifts, rotating two or three days on with two or three days off. This flexibility allows individuals to pursue hobbies, travel, and spend time with their families. As Vanessa, a nurse-practitioner who works in a California veterans' hospital, explains on the US Department of Veterans Affairs website, "My flexible work schedule has been very important to me, as I am active with my children's school."

Varying Educational Levels

Yet another advantage is that the health care industry employs people with varying educational levels. This makes it easy for individuals to find a career that fits their educational plans. Some health care careers, such as surgeon, anesthesiologist, or orthodontist, require more than ten years of specialized education and training beyond high school. Other positions require a master's, bachelor's, or associate's degree. But many jobs in this sector require a year or less of specialized training to become a licensed professional. This means that candidates with limited financial resources can start

Great Jobs in Health Care

Occupation	Minimum Educational Requirement	2017 Median Pay
Athletic trainer	Bachelor's degree	$46,630
Chiropractor	Doctoral or professional degree	$68,640
Dental hygienist	Associate's degree	$74,070
Dentist	Doctoral or professional degree	$158,120
EMT and paramedic	Postsecondary nondegree award, license	$33,380
Home health aide and personal care aide	High school diploma or equivalent	$23,130
Medical records and health care information technician	Postsecondary nondegree award	$39,180
Optician	High school diploma or equivalent	$36,250
Phlebotomist	Postsecondary nondegree award	$33,670
Physician and surgeon	Doctoral or professional degree	$208,000
Social worker	Bachelor's degree	$47,980

Source: Bureau of Labor Statistics, *Occupational Outlook Handbook*, 2018. www.bls.gov.

earning a living sooner. In addition, some jobs, such as personal care aides, medical secretaries, and hospital orderlies, provide high school graduates with on-the-job training.

Those who do receive specialized education and training beyond high school do not spend all of their time on academic studies. They receive hands-on learning opportunities in classrooms, laboratories, hospitals, and clinics. And there are ample opportunities for advancement. Many health care facilities offer employees specialized training and reimbursement for educational expenses so that individuals can advance in their chosen field.

Despite all these benefits, there is no doubt that the work of health care professionals can be physically, mentally, and emotionally challenging. They witness pain, suffering, and death; are exposed to blood-borne and infectious diseases; and often have to deal with frightened or discouraged patients. But most say the rewards outweigh the negatives. As Pasquini explains, "You get to help people every day and get paid to do it. . . . What an amazing experience!"

Dental Hygienist

What Does a Dental Hygienist Do?

Dental hygienists administer preventive dental procedures that help people ward off tooth decay, gum disease, and other oral health problems. They work under a dentist's supervision. Much of their time is spent cleaning deposits and stains from patients' teeth and gums. They use manual, power, and ultrasonic tools to remove hardened plaque that can cause gum disease and to get rid of stains on teeth. As part of the cleaning, they may apply fluoride and sealants that help protect teeth from tooth decay. What they do improves not only patients' dental health but their appearance and self-confidence as well. In an interview on the American Dental Education Association's website, Michigan dental hygienist Muntather Alameedi explains, "I had always received compliments about my smile, which had given me confidence growing up. The idea that just a smile could instill confidence led me to explore dental hygiene and my desire to help others have smiles just as healthy as mine."

Cleaning teeth is only part of a dental hygienist's job. When a patient visits a dental hygienist, the first thing the dental hygienist

At a Glance

Dental Hygienist

Minimum Educational Requirements
Associate's degree

Personal Qualities
Good manual dexterity, good interpersonal skills

Certification and Licensing
Dental hygienist license

Working Conditions
Indoors in dental offices

Salary Range
About $51,180 to $101,330

Number of Jobs
As of 2016, about 207,900

Future Outlook
20 percent growth, better than average

does is review the patient's medical history. The hygienist asks the patient about drug allergies, oral problems, and any recent illnesses and records the information in the patient's medical file. Next, dental hygienists examine the patient's teeth and gums. To check for tooth, gum, or jaw problems, they take, develop, and analyze dental X-rays. If they detect a problem, they report it to the dentist. If there are no problems that require care by the dentist, the hygienist cleans the patient's teeth. If the patient is sensitive to pain or requires a more extensive cleaning, the hygienist may administer a local anesthetic to numb the area, depending on state law.

As experts on oral hygiene, dental hygienists also educate patients on ways to improve and maintain their oral health. They explain the relationship between oral health and general health and between diet and oral health. They counsel patients on the best foods to eat to maintain oral health. They also instruct patients on how to brush and floss correctly, and they give advice on how to use and select toothbrushes, floss, and other dental devices. In an interview on the Dental Schools website, dental hygiene student Suzanne Hubbard explains, "What I love . . . most is when I have a patient sitting in front of me saying . . . 'I never knew that about my oral health, thank you so much for telling me!'"

How Do You Become a Dental Hygienist?

Education

To prepare for a career as a dental hygienist, in high school students should take classes in biology, chemistry, and health. Students need a basis in these subjects for dental hygiene training programs. Speech classes are also useful. Dental hygienists need good communication skills to explain procedures and instruct patients on dental health issues. Speech classes help individuals sharpen these skills. A psychology course is also helpful. Many people fear dental procedures. An understanding of human psychology helps dental hygienists put anxious patients at ease.

An associate's degree or a certificate from an accredited dental hygiene program is required for this profession. As of 2017, there were more than three hundred accredited dental hygiene programs offered in community colleges, technical schools, and universities in the United States. These programs usually require candidates to complete eighty-six credit hours and take two to three years to complete. Course work includes instruction in physiology, chemistry, nutrition, speech, English, and psychology, as well as classes specific to this career field, such as dental anatomy, oral and gum disease, X-ray technology, and medical ethics.

Hands-on training in laboratory classes teaches students how to use and care for a variety of dental tools. Training also includes extensive clinical practice under the supervision of experienced dental professionals. Hubbard describes her experience: "I like many aspects about my hygiene education; the fact that I will be competent in my skills before leaving the program is a positive. . . . The hands on phase is my favorite part of the education. . . . I see patients two days a week."

Certification and Licensing

Dental hygienists must be licensed. Licensing requirements vary by state. Generally, candidates must graduate from an accredited dental hygiene program and successfully complete a written exam, which usually lasts about eight hours. It is administered by the American Dental Association's Joint Commission on National Dental Examinations. Candidates must also pass a clinical exam administered by a state agency. Some states also require candidates to pass an exam on the legal aspects of dental hygiene practice.

Volunteer Work and Internships

Individuals interested in a career in dental hygiene can do a number of things to learn more about the field. Some dental practices hire part-time help to handle clerical duties. Taking on such a position is one good way for candidates to interact with dental hygienists and see what they do on a daily basis. Volunteering in a public health or school dental clinic provides a similar experience. Some dental hygienists will allow individuals interested in this career to follow and observe them as they work for a day or more. Individuals can also volunteer to instruct youth groups in proper brushing and flossing techniques, which is a good way to practice educating patients about oral health.

Skills and Personality

The mouth is a small area to work in. Good manual dexterity and eye-hand coordination helps dental hygienists successfully do their job. Without these traits, hygienists might inadvertently poke a sensitive spot in a patient's mouth, causing the patient unnecessary discomfort. These characteristics also help these professionals successfully use delicate tools.

Being physically fit is vital. Dental hygienists are on their feet much of the day. They bend over patients, twist their bodies while administering dental procedures, and work with their hands a lot. Not surprisingly, people with good physical stamina who enjoy working with their hands are often drawn to this profession.

Since a big part of their job involves interacting with others, dental hygienists should enjoy being around people and have good interpersonal and communication skills. These health care professionals may care for more than ten patients a day, and they regularly interact with the dentist and other dental office personnel. Individuals who like working with others and can communicate effectively do best under these circumstances.

Being patient, calm, and understanding are other essential traits that are needed in this profession. Many people are uneasy about dental procedures. Treating patients with compassion helps win their trust. In a February 2017 article in *RDH*, a magazine for dental professionals, Indiana dental hygienist Amber Metro-Sanchez writes, "Being a dental hygienist gives me a chance to change lives for the better. I'm given an opportunity to treat people with empathy and caring in order to build a founda-

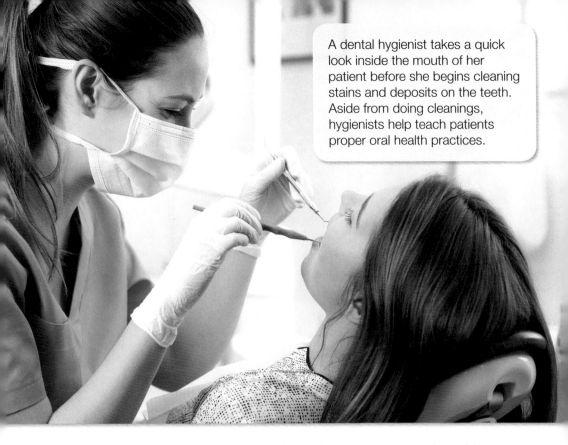

A dental hygienist takes a quick look inside the mouth of her patient before she begins cleaning stains and deposits on the teeth. Aside from doing cleanings, hygienists help teach patients proper oral health practices.

tion of trust. I can help scared patients become more relaxed in the dental office, and my ultimate success is when I have a patient who can't wait to come back." Indeed, it is not unusual for these personable professionals to come to know their patients well and develop long-term relationships with them.

On the Job

Employers

According to the Bureau of Labor Statistics (BLS), 95 percent of dental hygienists work in the offices of dentists. Others are employed by the military as commissioned officers who provide dental care to troops on military bases. Some work for federal, state, and local agencies in places like veterans' hospitals, public health clinics, schools, and prisons. Still others are employed in private hospitals, nursing homes, extended care facilities, and physicians' offices.

Working Conditions

Most dental hygienists work in clean, well-lit medical facilities. The BLS reports that 50 percent work part time. Full-time hygienists typically work a standard five-day, forty-hour week. Due to the nature of their work, dental hygienists face some occupational hazards. Working inside patients' mouths puts them in very close contact with their patients. They risk being exposed to blood-borne and infectious diseases. Frequent hand washing and wearing personal protective equipment such as safety glasses, gloves, and masks helps protect them. It also helps protect patients from contact with harmful germs.

In addition, because they perform repetitive motions with their hands and wrists and stand and bend for hours, it is common for dental hygienists to deal with musculoskeletal conditions like carpal tunnel syndrome and lower back pain. As Metro-Sanchez writes:

> Our jobs are very difficult, mentally and physically, and I could not imagine being a hygienist without being totally committed to my job every day. . . . And, of course, the ever-present reality of dealing with musculoskeletal injuries and pain is something nearly every hygienist has to face at some point. . . . There are many reasons why dental hygiene may not be the career of choice for everyone, but it is the career of choice for me.

Earnings

Dental hygienists' wages vary according to their experience, employer, and location. The BLS reports that as of May 2017, the median annual salary for this career was $74,070. The lowest-paid 10 percent of these professionals earned less than $51,180, while the highest-paid 10 percent earned more than $101,330. Average annual salaries are highest in the following states: Alaska, $107,190; California, $97,420; Washington, $91,070; and New Mexico, $89,740. Approximately 50 percent of dental hygienists receive employee benefits such as health insurance, sick leave, and paid vacation. Full-time workers are more likely to receive these benefits than part-time dental hygienists.

Opportunities for Advancement

Experienced dental hygienists employed in large dental practices may advance to an administrative position in which they supervise other hygienists and dental assistants. Obtaining a bachelor's or master's degree opens up other career opportunities. Dental hygienists with a bachelor's or master's degree can become classroom and/or clinical instructors in dental hygiene training programs. They can also move into oral health research positions.

What Is the Future Outlook for Dental Hygienists?

The BLS predicts that employment opportunities for dental hygienists will increase by 20 percent through 2026. This is much faster than the predicted average for all employment during this time. Much of this growth is due to an aging population that will need more dental care to maintain their teeth. A growing number of studies linking oral health to general health are also increasing demand for the services of dental hygienists. However, the number of graduates from dental hygiene programs is also growing, resulting in more competition for these jobs. Competition for jobs will vary by location. According to the BLS, employment opportunities will be best in rural areas where patients need dental care but have limited access to it.

Find Out More

American Dental Association (ADA)
211 E. Chicago Ave.
Chicago, IL 60611
website: www.ada.org

The ADA is the largest dental association in the United States. It provides information about a career as a dental hygienist. This includes a job description, advantages of this field, education and training requirements, licensure information, job opportunities, a video, and a list of further resources to contact.

American Dental Education Association (ADEA)
655 K St. NW, Suite 800
Washington, DC 20001
website: www.adea.org

The ADEA is an association whose members consist of students and faculty members of dental schools and other dental training programs, including dental hygienist training programs. It offers information about a career in dental hygiene and dental hygiene training programs.

American Dental Hygienist Association (ADHA)
444 N. Michigan Ave., Suite 400
Chicago, IL 60611
website: www.adha.org

The ADHA is a professional association that supports and represents dental hygienists and dental hygiene students. It provides a wealth of information about a career in dental hygiene.

National Dental Hygienists Association (NDHA)
website: www.NDHAonline.org

The NDHA promotes dental hygiene as a career for African Americans and other minorities. It offers scholarship information for students and information about career opportunities. It also publishes a newsletter and sponsors an annual conference.

Diagnostic Medical Sonographer

At a Glance

Diagnostic Medical Sonographer

Minimum Educational Requirements
Postsecondary training program

Personal Qualities
Enjoys working with people, good technical skills

Certification and Licensing
Certification required by most employers

Working Conditions
Indoors in health care facilities

Salary Range
About $50,760 to $99,840

Number of Jobs
As of 2016, about 122,300

Job Outlook
23 percent growth, better than average

What Does a Diagnostic Medical Sonographer Do?

Diagnostic medical sonographers, or sonographers, use ultrasound imaging technology to create and interpret images of internal body structures or, in the case of pregnancy, images of a developing fetus in the womb. By viewing these images, health care professionals can monitor and assess the development and position of a fetus, as well as establish the presence of multiple fetuses. These images are also instrumental in the detection and diagnosis of high-risk pregnancies, women's health issues, cancer, arterial blockages, and heart defects. As Texas diagnostic medical sonographer Christy N. Baez explains on the College of Health Care Professions blog, "The images I take help to diagnose, treat, and cure many people with diseases or life threatening illnesses. . . . Doctors depend on my finding to make their impressions [diagnoses]. People's lives are dependent on the images that I take. . . . I enjoy the variety of things that I scan all throughout the day such as infant brains, body tissues, blood vessels, or surgical procedures."

When sonographers work with a patient, the first thing they do is position the patient on an examining table so that the patient's body is at the best angle for imaging. Next, they rub gel on the skin that covers the internal area to be imaged. The gel allows high-frequency sound waves to be carried below the surface of the patient's skin. The sound waves are transmitted through a handheld medical device known as a transducer, which sonographers move over the area being studied. The sound waves reflect off the scanned area and are sent to a computer, which transforms the reflected waves into an image that is displayed on a monitor. To ensure that the image is clear and accurate, sonographers watch the monitor while administering the scan and make adjustments to the equipment if there is a problem. Once a good image is created, sonographers analyze it, looking for abnormalities, and prepare a written report for physicians based on their findings.

Sonographers usually specialize in imaging one or more specific areas of the body or a specific group of people. For instance, abdominal sonographers focus on internal structures within the abdominal cavity. Vascular sonographers scan blood vessels. Cardiac sonographers, or echocardiographers, take images of the heart. Musculoskeletal sonographers concentrate on muscles, tendons, ligaments, and joints. Neurological sonographers focus on the brain and nervous system, while breast sonographers scan breast tissue in order to identify the presence of cysts or tumors. Some sonographers concentrate on imaging infants and children. They are known as pediatric sonographers. Others, known as obstetrical and gynecological (OB/GYN) sonographers, scan the female reproductive system, including developing fetuses. This is diagnostic medical sonographer Sandra McKnight's specialty. In an interview on the Ultrasound Schools Info website, she explains, "I specialize in OB/GYN sonography and spend my days performing pelvic scans . . . and fetal scans at every gestational age. . . . It's an incredible experience to see your child [developing fetus] for the first time; it's an honor to share that experience with you as a sonographer."

How Do You Become a Diagnostic Medical Sonographer?

Education

It takes skill and knowledge to be a diagnostic medical sonographer. To prepare for a career as a sonographer, high school students should take classes in biology, algebra, and physics. A background in biology helps individuals understand human anatomy, while an understanding of physics and algebra are needed to solve problems related to the physical principles of sound. Plus, general physics and algebra are usually a prerequisite for admission to sonography programs. Technology classes are important, too. Sonographers must be comfortable working with sophisticated computerized equipment. Having good computer skills helps candidates learn to operate this equipment.

English and speech classes are also useful. Sonographers need to be able to communicate effectively. They should be able to discuss procedures with patients and give them clear instructions during the procedure. They also use communication skills to prepare written reports explaining their findings for other medical professionals.

High school graduates have three options to train for this career field. They can earn a certificate of completion from an accredited sonography program at a technical institute, which usually takes at least one year of postsecondary training. Or they can earn an associate's degree from an accredited sonography program at a community college, which takes two years to complete and is the most popular method. They can also enter the field with a bachelor's degree in an accredited sonography program from a four-year college.

Course work includes classes in anatomy, physiology, and sonographic physics, as well as classes that focus on operating ultrasound instruments, imaging different body parts, and the various specialty tracks. Hands-on laboratory practice is part of the curriculum. As Terrie Ciez, the program coordinator of the Diagnostic Medical Imaging Sonography Program at the College of DuPage in Glen Ellyn, Illinois, told the editors of the book *What Can I Do Now? Health Care*, "Students actually scan one another in order to learn how to identify normal and abnormal structures and anatomy and then be able to understand the pathology of various organs."

Students also get the chance to practice their imaging skills on patients under the guidance of an experienced sonographer. They usually rotate through different hospitals and medical facilities so that they get a broad range of experiences.

Certification and Licensing

Most employers require diagnostic medical sonographers to be registered. To become a registered diagnostic medical sonographer (RDMS), candidates must have graduated from an accredited diagnostic medical sonography program and pass an exam covering general sonography principles and instrumentation, an exam covering a specialty area of the candidate's choice, and a physics exam. The American Registry for Diagnostic Medical Sonographers administers the tests and awards certification. Candidates can earn additional credentials by successfully completing exams in multiple specialty areas.

Volunteer Work and Internships

Clinical practice in a sonography program serves as an internship. Before entering a sonography program, individuals can learn more about this field by following a registered sonographer through a workday. They can also learn more about sonography by volunteering to be a practice patient in a sonography training program. Since ultrasound technology does not emit harmful radiation, serving as a practice patient is not dangerous.

Skills and Personality

Sonographers need to be fit and strong. They are on their feet almost all day and have to help patients on and off examining tables. Additionally, they must be able to push ultrasound equipment that weighs about 50 pounds (22.7 kg) around hospitals. They need good vision and eye-hand coordination, too. These characteristics help sonographers effectively position and move the transducer while making adjustments in the scanning process in response to the images they see on the monitor.

Being technically adept and detail oriented are other important traits that help these professionals succeed in their careers. Sonographers must be comfortable working with and skilled in using complex equipment. While administering scans and analyzing images, they need to pay very careful attention to detail. Differences in normal and abnormal tissue can be very subtle. Missing an abnormality or mistaking normal tissue for abnormal tissue can have a dire effect on a patient's life.

Having good interpersonal skills is also valuable. To best serve patients that may be scared or in pain, sonographers need to be compassionate and kind. Good communication skills are vital, too. Sonographers interact with patients, patients' families, physicians, and coworkers. They must be able to communicate effectively with these people both orally and in writing.

In addition, sonographers should be good problem solvers. They use this skill in figuring out how to get the clearest images, as well as in determining how what they see in an image corresponds to a patient's symptoms. In an interview on the Ultrasound Technician Center website, Minnesota diagnostic medical sonographer Diane Harrison explains, "You're like the sleuth that comes in and figures out what is happening with this patient. You are looking through their organs and trying to figure out how what you are seeing comes into play with their symptoms. You are trying to help their Dr. figure that part of the puzzle out and help them to get better."

On the Job

Employers

Hospitals are the principal employer of sonographers. Sonographers also work in physicians' offices, imaging centers, and outpatient facilities. Some are employed in research facilities, while others work in educational institutions where they instruct sonography students. Sonographers also serve in the military.

Working Conditions

Sonographers work directly with patients in clean medical facilities. They often administer scans in dimly lit rooms. Dim lighting makes it easier to view the images on the monitor. They also perform procedures at patients' bedsides. Most work a five-day, forty-hour week. Part-time work is an option, too. The work hours of those employed in hospitals may include weekends, nights, holidays, and on-call hours. When on call, sonographers must be prepared to report to the hospital at any time. Some sonographers work twelve-hour alternating shifts with three or four days off per week.

Because this job is physically demanding and sonographers often perform repetitive and awkward motions in their work, many sonographers report musculoskeletal pain at some time in their career. Despite the risk of pain or injury, this profession ranked second in *U.S. News & World Report*'s 2018 ranking of the best health care support jobs and twenty-sixth in its ranking of the one hundred best jobs overall.

Earnings

The Bureau of Labor Statistics (BLS) reports that as of May 2017, the median annual salary for diagnostic medical sonographers was $71,410. The lowest-paid 10 percent of these professionals earned less than $50,760, while the highest-paid 10 percent earned more than $99,840. Earnings are usually based on an individual's experience, credentials, education level, employer, and location. Individuals with the most experience on the job, higher levels of education, and certification in multiple specialties receive the highest compensation. In addition to their wages, most sonographers receive generous employee benefits that typically include health insurance, a retirement plan, and paid sick and vacation days.

Opportunities for Advancement

Holding multiple certificates broadens a sonographer's area of expertise, which boosts employment prospects and enhances opportunities for advancement. Sonographers with extensive experience can become clinical supervisors or hospital ultrasound department administrators. Those with a bachelor's degree can teach in sonography training programs or work in research.

What Is the Future Outlook for Diagnostic Medical Sonographers?

According to the BLS, employment opportunities for diagnostic medical sonographers are expected to grow by 23 percent through 2026. This is much faster than the predicted average for all employment growth in the same period. Demand is projected to be greatest for individuals certified in more than one specialty area.

Find Out More

American Institute of Ultrasound in Medicine (AIUM)
14750 Sweitzer Ln., Suite 100
Laurel, MD 20707
website: www.aium.org

The AIUM is a professional organization dedicated to the field of ultrasound. It offers lots of information about various ultrasound specialties, including online lectures and webinars, as well as providing practice exams for different specialty credentials.

American Registry for Diagnostic Medical Sonographers (ARDMS)
1401 Rockville Pike, Suite 600
Rockville, MD 20852
website: www.ardms.org

The ARDMS administers exams and awards credentials in areas of ultrasound. Candidates can register for exams on the website. The ARDMS also provides information about careers in sonography and the exams.

Society of Diagnostic Medical Sonographers
2745 Dallas Pkwy.
Plano, TX 75092
website: www.sdms.org

The Society of Diagnostic Medical Sonographers is a network of sonographers, students, educators, and other health care providers interested in sonography. It provides lots of information about this career field, training programs, certification, and a job board.

Ultrasound Schools Info
website: www.ultrasoundschoolsinfo.com

This website provides a comprehensive database of accredited diagnostic medical sonographer programs. It also gives information about the career, specializations, how ultrasound works, and salaries and provides interviews with sonographers.

Massage Therapist

Massage therapists are health care professionals who, through touch, manipulate a client's muscles and soft tissues to improve the client's physical health and overall well-being. Research indicates that massage therapy, which is considered to be a nontraditional alternative form of health care, has many health benefits. In an interview on the website of College of Lake County, Rick Smith, the founder of Illinois's Parkland College massage therapy program, explains:

> In only a few sessions massage therapy can relieve, to one degree or another, physical stress and discomfort, muscular pain, emotional stress and tension, limited range of motion, and that overall feeling of malaise. And all without drugs or invasive procedures. Massage is a natural way to provide relief and comfort to someone. . . . When clients leave my office, both they and I feel better.

At a Glance

Massage Therapist

Minimum Educational Requirements
Postsecondary nondegree program

Personal Qualities
Physical strength and stamina, good interpersonal skills

Certification and Licensing
Massage therapist license

Working Conditions
Indoors, primarily in spas and resorts, hospitals and wellness centers, offices of other health care professionals, clients' homes, and private practices

Salary Range
About $20,300 to $77,470

Number of Jobs
As of 2016, about 160,300

Future Outlook
26 percent growth, better than average

When administering a massage, massage therapists begin by creating a relaxing atmosphere. They may dim the lights and play calming music. Using oil to lubricate the client's skin and reduce friction, they rub the client's skin and underlying muscles. They apply varying pressure, depending on the individual's particular health issues and the type of massage.

There are different types of massage, and most therapists specialize in more than one type. Some massage therapists also specialize in treating specific age groups, like children or the elderly. Every client has unique needs. Some are in pain; others need to unwind; some want to hasten the rehabilitation of a sports injury, among other things. Massage therapists customize the length, intensity, and kind of massage based on the person's physical condition, age, and particular health issues. "I always use a questionnaire completed by the client to assess his or her physical or emotional state prior to the massage. Then I decide what kind of bodywork to do," massage therapist Donda Sternberg explains in an interview on the Natural Healers website.

Between massage sessions, therapists work on scheduling, billing, and updating the files they keep on their clients. They also get ready for their next session. This involves refreshing the room, sanitizing the massage table, and changing the linens. In an interview on CareerColleges.com, Michigan health spa massage therapist Julie Azzopardi describes a typical day:

A typical day for me, on a Saturday for example, is that I am in (to work) at 10 in the morning. If I have a 10 a.m. client, then I am usually there a half hour beforehand, so I can get the room ready. You get a half hour between clients to turn around the table. . . . So if I have a 10 a.m. (client), that could go from 10 a.m. to 11 a.m. and then my next one could come in at 11:30 a.m. and be there until 12:30 p.m. I could have as many as four clients a day or as little as two, and client sessions last as short as a half hour and as long as an hour and a half.

How Do You Become a Massage Therapist?

Education

After earning a high school diploma, the best way to become a massage therapist is by attending an accredited massage therapy program in which candidates receive approximately five hundred hours of state-recognized training. Most programs take less than one year to complete and are offered in massage therapy schools, vocational institutes, and community colleges.

To prepare for a career as a massage therapist, high school students should take classes in biology (or anatomy, if it is offered) so that they have a basic understanding of the human body. Speech classes help candidates develop the communication skills that they will need to explain procedures to their clients. Classes in business and marketing benefit prospective therapists who hope to start their own practice in the future.

Postsecondary programs combine classroom instruction with hands-on practice and field experience. Students are instructed in physiology, anatomy, kinesiology (the scientific study of human movement), medical ethics, assessment of patients' needs, and different massage techniques. Classroom instruction is reinforced by hands-on practice in an on-site massage facility or through an internship program. In either case, students are given the opportunity to massage clients under the supervision of experienced practitioners.

Certification and Licensing

Requirements for certification and licensing vary by state and municipality. According to the Bureau of Labor Statistics (BLS), forty-five states and the District of Columbia have laws regulating massage therapy. Depending on the state, typical requirements include graduation from an accredited training program and the successful completion of a state licensing exam. Individuals can become nationally board certified by passing an exam administered by the National Certification Board for Therapeutic Massage and Bodywork. Having national board certification is prestigious. It can help practitioners grow their client base and advance their careers.

Volunteer Work and Internships

One way individuals can learn more about this profession is by getting a massage at a massage therapy school's on-site massage facility. Individuals can talk to student practitioners about their training and observe them as they practice their art. Following a massage therapist through a workday is another good way to learn more about massage therapy.

Massage therapy students have a variety of options for participating in an internship. Most commonly, massage therapy schools have on-site massage facilities that are open to the public. As part of their studies, students administer massages in these facilities for a set number of hours determined by the school. This serves as an internship. In other cases, massage therapy programs place student interns in medical facilities, spas, sports rehabilitation clinics, and wellness centers. As with on-site facilities, student interns train in these facilities for a set number of hours.

Skills and Personality

This is a physically challenging career. Massage therapists usually administer multiple massages on any given day. While administering a massage, they stand on their feet and exert force with their hands, arms, and shoulders to manipulate a client's muscles. Therefore, they should be physically fit, have strength and lots of stamina, and like working with their hands.

Massage therapists come into very close contact with their clients. They should be comfortable touching others and like working with people. Personable individuals who can put clients at ease and be empathetic to their needs build trust with their clients. This helps practitioners expand their client base. Strong communication and listening skills are also essential. Therapists must be able to communicate clearly and effectively with their clients. And, in order to customize massage sessions to suit each person's individual needs, therapists must listen carefully as their clients describe their health issues.

Being a good businessperson is also helpful, especially for self-employed massage therapists. These individuals must be skilled

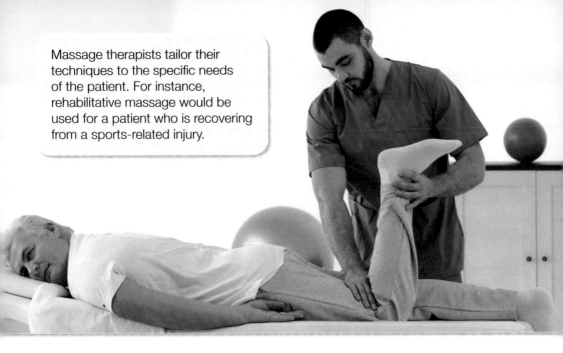

Massage therapists tailor their techniques to the specific needs of the patient. For instance, rehabilitative massage would be used for a patient who is recovering from a sports-related injury.

at managing their time, handling financial matters, and marketing themselves. Moreover, in order to increase their client base, even salaried massage therapists are expected to market themselves. As Azzopardi explains, "Even though the spa I work at does market (itself), to get the repeat clients I want . . . I do need to market myself."

On the Job

Employers
Approximately 39 percent of all massage therapists are self-employed. They work out of offices in their homes, work in private studios, or travel to their clients' homes or offices to administer a massage. Other massage therapists work in physicians' and chiropractors' offices, nursing homes, sports medicine facilities, and wellness centers. Some work in spas, salons, fitness centers, and yoga studios. Still others work in hotels, resorts, and cruise ships. Sports teams employ massage therapists, too.

Working Conditions
Working conditions vary, depending on the employer. Most massage therapists work in clean, dimly lit rooms with soothing music playing softly in the background. Some self-employed massage therapists

spend a good part of their day traveling to and from patients' homes or offices. These individuals provide their own massage table, linens, and body oils, which they transport, load, and unload. Self-employed practitioners who work out of home offices or private studios do not travel, but they, too, provide their own supplies.

Work hours are usually flexible. Most massage therapists see clients by appointment, so their work schedule varies from day to day. Many work evenings and weekends to suit their clients' schedules. About half of all massage therapists work part time. Since this job is very physically demanding, many practitioners cannot administer massages eight hours per day, five days per week. In order to avoid injuries, they try to space their appointments so that they have time to rest between sessions. Still, because they perform repetitive motions with their arms, hands, and wrists and stand and bend for hours, many practitioners deal with lower back pain and musculoskeletal issues. To avoid pain and injuries, massage therapists try to space their sessions, use good body mechanics, and trade massages with other therapists. Azzopardi explains, "We do trades amongst our other colleagues in the spa. I have been trying to get [massages] as frequently as I can—usually about once a week to once every other week. But I've been really fortunate in the sense that I don't overburden myself. I do really try to keep that balance. If I am not able to do massages, I am able to block my schedule off. (The job) is flexible." Indeed, the flexibility of being able to set their own work hours and being able to choose among a variety of work environments makes this a very appealing profession for many individuals.

Earnings

The BLS reports that the median wage for massage therapists in 2017 was $39,900; the lowest-paid 10 percent of massage therapists earned less than $20,300 and the highest-paid 10 percent earned more than $77,470. Earnings depend on the number of hours therapists work, the employer, the employer's location, and the massage therapist's level of experience, education, number of clients, and ability to administer different types of massage. In addition to their wages, most massage therapists earn tips. Full-time salaried massage therapists usually receive employee benefits such as health insurance, free massages, paid vacation and sick days, and a retirement plan. Part-time and self-employed professionals usually do not receive any employee benefits.

Opportunities for Advancement

Some massage therapists begin their careers as salaried employees in a health or wellness facility, salon, or small spa. Once they gain experience and a client base, they often open their own massage therapy practice. Self-employed massage therapists increase their earnings by building up a large, repeat client base. As their practice grows, they may employ other massage therapists whom they supervise.

Experienced massage therapists who are adept at multiple types of massage can also gain employment in posh destination spas that typically offer generous wages and benefits in order to attract the most-skilled practitioners. They can also advance to administrative positions as spa directors and managers.

What Is the Future Outlook for Massage Therapists?

The BLS predicts that employment opportunities for massage therapists will increase by 26 percent through 2026, which is much higher than the average for all occupations. This growth is due to the growing awareness and acceptance by health care professionals and the general public of the value of massage.

Find Out More

American Massage Therapy Association (AMTA)
500 Davis St., Suite 900
Evanston, IL 60201
website: www.amtamassage.org

The AMTA is a professional association of massage therapists and massage therapy students. Its website offers career and scholarship information and provides online courses. The association also publishes a massage therapy journal and a monthly newsletter for massage therapy students.

Associated Bodyworks and Massage Professionals (ABMP)
25188 Genesee Trail Rd., Suite 200
Golden, CO 80401
e-mail: expectmore@abmp.com
website: www.abmp.com

The ABMP is a professional association of massage therapists and massage therapy students and educators. It offers free massage therapy technique videos, study guides, practice tests for licensing and certification, and tips on creating a website for self-marketing.

Commission on Massage Therapy Accreditation
2101 Wilson Blvd., Suite 302
Arlington, VA 22201
e-mail: info@comta.org
website: www.comta.org

This organization accredits massage therapy programs. It provides a list of all accredited programs and schools in the United States on its website, as well as information about the curriculum in these programs. It also offers grants.

Massage Therapy Foundation
500 Davis St., Suite 950
Evanston, IL 60201
website: http://massagetherapyfoundation.org

This foundation supports scientific research on therapeutic massage. It was founded by the American Massage Therapy Association, but the two organizations are separate entities. It publishes an academic journal and offers research grants, research findings, e-books, podcasts, and a blog.

Nurse-Midwife

Nurse-midwives are advanced-practice nurses. This means that they are registered nurses who have a master's degree and specialized training and credentials, which qualifies them to work autonomously (without a physician's supervision) in most states. There are different types of advanced-practice nurses. Nurse-midwives specialize in women's sexual and reproductive health issues with a focus on pregnancy, labor and delivery, postpartum care, and newborn care.

In the past, nurse-midwives were almost always female. But that is no longer the case. Modern nurse-midwives are both male and female. These health care professionals have many responsibilities. They examine, monitor, and record the progress of expectant mothers and developing fetuses during the course of pregnancy. They also counsel expectant mothers and their families about what to expect during pregnancy, labor, and delivery, as well as instruct them about proper nutrition, breastfeeding, and infant care. Once patients go into labor, nurse-midwives are present throughout the birthing process to supervise and assist with labor and delivery.

At a Glance

Nurse-Midwife

Minimum Educational Requirements
Master's degree

Personal Qualities
Good critical-thinking skills, good interpersonal skills

Certification and Licensing
Registered nurse license, national certification

Working Conditions
Indoors in a health care facility

Salary Range
About $76,830 to $180,460

Number of Jobs
As of 2016, about 6,500

Future Job Outlook
21 percent growth, better than average

Nurse-midwives usually work with healthy women who are at low risk for complications during pregnancy or childbirth. However, they are trained to deal with complications such as hemorrhaging, twin and multiple births, or births in which the baby is in the wrong position. They work as a team with expectant mothers. Together they come up with a plan for the birthing process that best suits each patient's particular needs and desires, including the best options for managing labor pain. Most nurse-midwives are skilled in using a variety of methods to make patients more comfortable during delivery. As nurse-midwife Shelly Boone explains in an article posted on the Huntington County (Indiana) Chamber of Commerce website:

> Whether you wish to use relaxation techniques or movement during labor—or try IV, epidural, or other medications—the midwife can work with you to help meet your desired approach to birth. . . . The mom calls the shots. And it's a team effort. It's my job to supervise a normal, healthy pregnancy and delivery, and to recognize when/if there is something abnormal. It's about being present, and guiding the mom to do the job her body needs her to do.

In addition to providing care for pregnant women, many nurse-midwives also provide gynecological care, well-woman exams, primary health care, and family planning services for women of all ages. Because they are advanced-practice nurses they are able to prescribe medication, order medical tests, administer vaccinations, and perform screening tests. According to Boone, "Midwife, means 'with woman.' And I'm here to walk beside my patients no matter what stage of life they're in."

How Do You Become a Nurse-Midwife?

Education
In order to become a nurse-midwife, candidates must earn a bachelor's degree in nursing and a master's degree in midwifery.

It typically takes two years of education beyond a bachelor's degree, or a total of six years of education beyond high school, to enter this career field.

To prepare for a career as a nurse-midwife, high school students should take classes in health, biology, and chemistry. A strong science background is needed for challenging undergraduate and graduate course work. Admission into both undergraduate nursing programs and graduate-level midwifery programs is competitive. Students should try to maintain a high grade point average to improve their chances of admission.

There are approximately forty accredited midwifery programs in the United States. Since graduate-level course work builds on what students learned in undergraduate nursing programs and in clinical practice, candidates are required to be registered nurses with a minimum of one year of clinical experience. Graduate-level classes focus on areas such as women's health, pregnancy, fetal development, midwifery care during labor, and newborn care. Students also receive instruction in physiology, anatomy, pharmacology, and medical ethics, among other topics. Classroom instruction is combined with clinical experience in hospitals and birthing centers, which gives candidates the opportunity to work with expectant mothers under the supervision of experienced certified nurse-midwives. Students usually accrue from seven hundred to one thousand hours of clinical experience by the time they graduate.

Certification and Licensing

Certification is required in most, but not all, states. Typically, nurse-midwives are required to have a registered nursing license, graduate from an accredited midwifery program, and successfully complete a national certification exam administered by the American Midwifery Certification Board.

Volunteer Work and Internships

Individuals interested in a career in midwifery can learn more about nursing and midwifery and experience what it is like to work with patients by volunteering at a woman's health clinic or the maternity ward of a hospital. Volunteers get to see how these facilities are run. They also have the opportunity to talk to nurse-midwives about their work. Following a nurse-midwife through a typical workday is another way individuals can see exactly what nurse-midwives do, experience various cases and situations, and gain a better understanding of the scope of the profession.

A number of international organizations and private companies offer opportunities for student midwives to do service projects and internships in medical facilities in Asia, Africa, the Caribbean, and Latin America. Participants get clinical experience while making a real contribution to women in need.

Skills and Personality

Nurse-midwives should have a strong foundation in nursing and be knowledgeable in all areas of women's health. Since they work as a team with patients and patients' families, they should have good interpersonal and communication skills. Pregnancy is an emotional and often stressful time for women. Having good interpersonal skills will help nurse-midwives build rapport and trust with their patients. Having good communication skills allows these professionals to clearly convey information to their patients, as well as to other health care professionals. And since their patients are likely to come from diverse backgrounds, nurse-midwives should be nonjudgmental and tolerant of patients with different values.

These professionals should also be observant and detail oriented. These skills allow them to successfully assess a patient's health and that of the fetus, noting even the smallest of changes. These skills help nurse-midwives detect the patient's spoken and unspoken needs, too. Staying calm under pressure and having good critical-thinking and problem-solving skills are also vital. The birthing process does not always proceed the way it should. Should problems arise, nurse-midwives have to make rapid decisions concerning the best course of action to take. Their decisions and actions permanently impact their patients and their families and can make the difference between life and death for mothers and babies.

In addition to these skills, nurse-midwives should be physically fit. Midwives stand, bend, twist, lift, and hold their bodies in fixed positions for long periods. In order to do their job effectively, they should be healthy and have lots of stamina. They also need good eye-hand coordination and steady hands to do their job effectively. As nurse-midwife and blogger Andrea Altomaro explains on the PBS website, "Our hands are our tools; from the technical skills of delivery and suturing to the act of gently wiping the brow of a laboring mother, or applying counter pressure on her lower back, the use of our hands is vital to our profession."

On the Job

Employers
The Bureau of Labor Statistics (BLS) estimates that nearly 50 percent of nurse-midwives in the United States are employed in physicians' offices. Nurse-midwives are also employed in a number of other settings, including hospitals, community health centers, women's health facilities, birthing centers, and educational institutions. Many nurse-midwives are self-employed.

Working Conditions
Most nurse-midwives work indoors in clean, well-lit health care facilities. Some nurse-midwives choose to work in refugee camps and/or health clinics in war-torn and developing nations. Working conditions in these sites can be quite primitive. Others attend births in patients' homes.

No matter where they work, nurse-midwives are on call to respond to patients who go into labor. Most work full time. Those who are employed by hospitals and other round-the-clock health care facilities often work in eight- to twelve-hour rotating shifts. They may work three or four days, including nights, holidays, and weekends, with three or four days off. Self-employed nurse-midwives set their own hours.

This is a physically taxing profession. It is not uncommon for nurse-midwives to experience musculoskeletal pain in their backs, hands, and wrists caused or exacerbated by their work. They are also at risk of exposure to blood-borne and infectious diseases. Yet despite these drawbacks, most nurse-midwives are satisfied with their career choice. As Kate, a British nurse-midwife explains on the Your Midwife Career website, "There is nothing more rewarding than being the first person to see a new baby making an appearance."

Earnings

The BLS reports that as of May 2017, the median annual wage for nurse-midwives was $100,590. It reports that the lowest-paid 10 percent earned less than $76,830, while the highest-paid 10 percent earned more than $180,460. Earnings vary by region and employer. Average wages are highest in the following states: California, $132,480; West Virginia, $126,260; Massachusetts, $119,700; New Jersey, $111,600; and Wisconsin, $109,280.

Salaried nurse-midwives usually receive paid benefits such as health insurance, a retirement plan, cell phone reimbursement, and paid sick and vacation days. Many medical facilities offer nurse-midwives generous sign-on bonuses and relocation assistance. Self-employed nurse-midwives do not receive employee benefits.

Opportunities for Advancement

This is not an entry-level career field. Nurse-midwives start their careers as registered nurses; after advanced training and clinical experience, they become nurse-midwives. Most start their midwife careers as salaried employees in hospitals, physicians' offices, birth centers, and other health care facilities. After gaining experience, some open independent or group practices with other nurse-midwives. Successful practices can be quite lucrative and give nurse-midwives the freedom to be their own boss and the flexibility to arrange their own employment conditions. Moreover, since nurse-midwives are advanced-practice nurses, by successfully completing a licensing exam, they can become a licensed nurse-practitioner. This qualifies them to perform many of the same medical services as a primary care physician. Holding dual licenses allows these professionals to expand their practices to include primary care for males and females of all ages.

Experienced nurse-midwives can also advance to administrative positions in hospital maternity wards, women's health facilities, and birthing centers. Others work as instructors in nursing and nurse-midwife training programs at colleges and universities. They can also work in research, pharmaceutical sales, and global health.

What Is the Future Outlook for Nurse-Midwives?

The BLS predicts that employment opportunities for nurse-midwives will increase by 21 percent through 2026. This is faster than the average growth rate for other professions. More individuals are turning to midwives as an increasing number of expectant mothers seek more personal and holistic care. Additionally, the growing expansion of most health insurance to include midwife care should also increase the demand for these professionals.

Find Out More

American College of Nurse-Midwives (ACNM)
8403 Colesville Rd., Suite 1550
Silver Spring, MD 20910
website: www.midwife.org

The ACNM is a professional organization that promotes midwifery education and research. It offers a wealth of information about this career field, including information about how high school students can best prepare for this profession.

American Midwifery Certification Board (AMCB)
849 International Dr., Suite 120
Linthicum, MD 21090
website: www.amcbmidwife.org

The AMCB is the national certifying organization for nurse-midwives. It provides information about the certifying exam, what nurse-midwives do, and women's health.

Midwife Career
e-mail: support@midwifecareer.com
website: www.midwifecareer.com

This British website provides information about this career field. It offers interviews with British nurse-midwives, information about midwifery education, and a blog.

RN to BSN
801 Congress St., Suite 400
Houston, TX 77002
website: www.rntobsn.org

This organization is made up of nurses, educators, and others committed to furthering nursing education. Its website provides information on all types of advanced-practice nursing careers, including nurse-midwife, as well as information about educational programs, scholarships, and certification.

Occupational Therapist

Occupational therapists (also known as OTs) help physically, mentally, emotionally, and developmentally disabled, injured, or ill people develop, improve, or recover the skills needed to perform everyday activities. These activities are known as *occupations*. Learning or relearning how to dress, bathe, or self-feed are just a few of these occupations. In an interview with the editors of the book *Hot Health Care Careers*, New Mexico OT Melissa Winkle explains, "When people work with occupational therapists they are able to return to doing something they have not been able to do for a period of time. Other clients learn how to do something that they have never been able to do before. . . . The goal is for them to become as independent as possible, or to regain their dignity and self-sufficiency."

Each patient's case is different. Upon meeting a new patient, the first thing an OT does is evaluate

At a Glance

Occupational Therapist

Minimum Educational Requirements
Master's degree

Personal Qualities
Good at motivating others, good communication skills

Certification and Licensing
Occupational therapist license

Working Conditions
Indoors in health care facilities or educational settings

Salary Range
About $54,560 to $120,440

Number of Jobs
As of 2016, about 130,400

Future Outlook
24 percent growth, better than average

that person's strengths, weaknesses, and capabilities. Then, based on this assessment and the patient's input about his or her specific needs and goals, the OT creates a customized care plan for that person. The focus is primarily on, but not limited to, developing and improving fine motor skills. OTs work with patients on self-care tasks such as personal hygiene, self-feeding, and grooming. They also work on the skills needed to write, use a computer, and prepare food, among other things. They use therapeutic activities such as games, physical exercises, and art activities to help patients achieve their goals. For instance, to improve manual dexterity, OTs might have individuals string beads or play with clay. They use computer and card games to improve the memory skills of people with brain-related issues.

This is not all these professionals do. As part of their duties, OTs visit patients' homes, where they identify household risks and help patients and their families modify their homes to make them safer and more accessible. Another part of an OT's job is helping individuals find and use ergonomic and adaptive tools that meet that person's specific needs. For example, an OT might help patients with limited use of their hands or feet acquire and learn to use a wheelchair that can be controlled with the patient's head. Similarly, OTs help patients locate and use ergonomic tools designed to improve dexterity. And, if appropriate adaptive equipment cannot be found, it is not unusual for creative OTs to craft simple tools themselves.

People in need of occupational therapy range from children to the elderly and have diverse health issues. OTs who go into general practice work with a wide range of patients. Or they can limit their practice to a particular area of occupational therapy. Specialties include pediatric, geriatric, mental health, and rehabilitation occupational therapy. Pediatric OTs work with children and adolescents who have developmental delays, learning disabilities, or conditions like cerebral palsy or autism. Geriatric OTs work with elderly individuals, who often have multiple health conditions that hamper their ability to function. Psychiatric OTs work with people with mental health issues. In this capacity, they may teach patients with anger issues relaxation techniques, among other things. Finally, rehabilitation OTs work with individuals recovering from an injury or a health condition like a stroke to help them regain or compensate for lost function.

How Do You Become an Occupational Therapist?

Education

To prepare for a career as an OT, high school students should take classes in biology, health, and psychology. Knowledge of the human body is essential to this field, while understanding human behavior helps OTs motivate reluctant patients. And since OTs must communicate with patients, patients' families, and other health care professionals, English and speech classes are helpful in developing good communication skills.

A master's degree is required to become an OT. Some universities offer a dual-degree program in occupational therapy, which allows students to earn a bachelor's and a master's degree in a total of five years. However, in most cases it takes two years beyond a bachelor's degree, or a total of six years of education beyond high school, to qualify for this career.

Graduate programs in occupational therapy admit students with a variety of college majors. Related majors that prepare candidates for a graduate-level program include occupational therapy, kinesiology, biology, psychology, and health science. Graduate-level classes focus on the skills and knowledge needed to succeed in this career. Course work includes classes in physiology, neuroscience, psychology, childhood development and disabilities, and rehabilitation methods, to name a few. As part of their training, students are required to do clinical fieldwork, which is similar to a medical internship. In this capacity, participants work with patients full-time for a minimum of twenty-four weeks under the supervision of an experienced OT.

Certification and Licensing

OTs must be certified. To become certified, candidates must graduate from an accredited occupational therapy program with a master's degree and pass a national written exam administered by the National Board for Certification in Occupational Therapy.

Candidates can obtain additional, specialty certification from the American Occupational Therapy Association. Specialty certification includes certification in pediatric, rehabilitation, geriatric, and psychiatric occupational therapy. Other specialty certification is available for individuals who want to provide OT services in schools; focus their practice on treating people with low vision; or help those with feeding, eating, or swallowing problems, among other areas.

Volunteer Work and Internships

Prospective OTs can gain firsthand knowledge about this profession and see whether this career suits their interests and abilities in a number of ways. For instance, volunteering to work with people with disabilities or working as a counselor in a camp for physically or mentally challenged children allows individuals to see whether they like working with the disabled. Volunteering in an occupational therapy department of a hospital, nursing home, or rehabilitation facility, and/or following an OT through a typical workday are other valuable experiences. These give individuals a chance to interact with OTs and learn more about what the job actually entails.

Skills and Personality

Successful OTs are personable and have good communication skills. These professionals spend a lot of time getting to know their patients and their goals and instructing them. These duties require that OTs be pleasant, good listeners, and able to explain things clearly.

Creativity, patience, compassion, and a positive attitude are also needed for this job. People undergoing occupational therapy can be easily frustrated and want to give up. If an activity is overwhelming for a patient, OTs must be able to come up with another method for that patient to master the goal. This may involve creating an entirely new activity or breaking down the task into smaller, more readily achievable activities. No matter the solution, OTs must be able to motivate the people they serve. Patience, understanding, and an upbeat demeanor go a long way in keeping patients on track. As OT and blogger Marlene Hampton explains on St. Catherine University's website, "The word I like best to describe my typical day as an inpatient rehabilitation occupational therapist is 'motivating.' As an occupational therapist, you are constantly motivating patients to achieve a greater level of independence. Meanwhile, your patients have a way of motivating you to strive to be the best you can be."

On the Job

Employers

OTs work in a variety of settings. They are employed by hospitals, mental health centers, rehabilitation facilities, and skilled nursing facilities. They also work in schools, group homes, the offices of other health care providers, and community health facilities. Some work for home health care agencies, while other OTs are self-employed. Some work for multiple employers or in more than one facility and travel from facility to facility. Some OTs work with patients in the patients' homes, which requires traveling between sessions.

Working Conditions

Most OTs work indoors in clean, well-lit health care facilities. Most work a five-day, forty-hour week, which may include evenings and weekends, depending on the employer. One out of three OTs work part time. Those who are self- employed set their own hours.

People in the profession face some health risks. Because OTs are in direct contact with their patients, they may be exposed to bodily fluids that can cause infectious diseases. This is especially a problem for OTs teaching or helping people regain toileting, self-feeding, and personal hygiene skills. Washing their hands frequently and sanitizing therapy equipment helps OTs protect themselves from germs. Muscle strain is another possible hazard of the job. OTs often have to lift or move patients, which puts them at risk for musculoskeletal injuries. In addition, this job can be emotionally challenging. OTs often work with frustrated individuals, who may take out their frustrations on their therapist. Sometimes, patients die due to illness. Such situations can be stressful for OTs and may cause some to become depressed.

Earnings

According to the Bureau of Labor Statistics (BLS), as of May 2017 the median annual salary for OTs was $83,200. The lowest-paid 10 percent of OTs earn less than $54,560, while the highest-paid 10 percent earn more than $120,440. Salaries depend on an individual's experience, education, and the type and location of the employer. As of May 2017, the BLS reported the following median salary for OTs by employer: skilled nursing facilities, $90,980; home health care services, $87,680; office of other health care providers, $85,190; hospitals, $83,369; and schools, $73,260. It reports the following states with the highest average wage for OTs: Nevada, $103,280; Texas, $95,430; and New Jersey, $94,100.

Opportunities for Advancement

With experience, OTs can advance to administrative positions supervising other OTs. Some experienced OTs go into private practice. Those with specialty certification are in demand and often command higher wages. Opportunities also exist for OTs to teach in colleges and universities, do research, or work in therapy product sales.

What Is the Future Outlook for Occupational Therapists?

The BLS predicts that employment opportunities for OTs will grow by 24 percent through 2026, which is much faster than average. High employment growth is attributed to an aging population. OTs will be needed to help senior citizens remain active and maintain their independence. OT services will also be in demand by Americans recovering from strokes and other health issues related to aging. The growing number of diagnoses of autism spectrum disorders may also mean more work for OTs. Job prospects will be best for individuals with multiple specialty certificates. Indeed, strong and growing employment opportunities were important reasons why Texas OT Joshua Springer chose this career. In an article on the OT Career Path website he explains: "Job security and availability was a top priority, and [I] found that occupational therapy is on the rise and will continue to be in demand for many years to come."

Find Out More

American Occupational Therapy Association (AOTA)
4720 Montgomery Lane, Suite 200
Bethesda, MD 20814
website: www.aota.org

The AOTA is a professional association that represents the interests of OTs, occupational therapy assistants, and occupational therapy students. It provides information about the profession, occupational therapy programs, scholarships, fieldwork, job resources, and certification.

National Board for Certification in Occupational Therapy (NBCOT)
12 S. Summit Ave., Suite 100
Gaithersburg, MD 20877
website: www.nbcot.org

The NBCOT certifies OTs. It offers information about exams, exam applications, study guides, and practice tests.

OT Career Path
website: www.otcareerpath.com

This website provides lots of information for students considering a career of occupational therapy. It offers information about the profession, a listing of accredited OT programs, licensing, salaries, and interviews with OTs.

OT Potential
website: www.otpotential.com

OT Potential is a website that provides information and resources for OTs, OT students, and people interested in occupational therapy. Among its offerings are blog posts, articles, tips on finding jobs, and links to publications.

Pediatrician

Pediatricians are physicians who specialize in the care and treatment of infants, children, and adolescents. These physicians are especially knowledgeable about common childhood health conditions like flu, ear infections, and whooping cough and the treatment of minor injuries, but they also provide care for young people with life-threatening conditions. Among their duties, they monitor patients' growth and development, conduct physical exams, diagnose illness, order and interpret medical tests, and prescribe medicine. They make referrals to and collaborate with other health care providers. They also counsel parents about childhood health and development. In an interview on the Cook Children's Health Care System website, Texas pediatrician Justin Smith explains, "I love walking into a room where mom has a list of questions (no, really). What that means is I am going to provide relevant answers and suggestions important to that family. . . . That's my reason for dedicating my practice to pediatrics. . . . I want to help you go through your own journey and make the best decisions for your family."

At a Glance

Pediatrician

Minimum Educational Requirements
Doctor of medicine or doctor of osteopathy degree

Personal Qualities
Enjoy working with children, observant

Certification and Licensing
Physician's license

Working Conditions
Indoors in a health care facility

Salary Range
About $82,670 to more than $208,000

Number of Jobs
As of 2017, about 28,990

Future Job Outlook
15 percent growth, better than average

It is common for pediatricians to treat young patients for at least a decade. Often, they treat multiple children in a family. As a result, many pediatricians get to know and develop a close relationship with their patients and their families. As one pediatrician told the editors of *Pediatrics 101*, a resource guide from the American Academy of Pediatrics (AAP), "When you're a general pediatrician you're a member of every family that you take care of. Would I recommend pediatrics? You bet your life!"

Pediatricians can choose to be general pediatricians, or they can limit their practice to one of many pediatric subspecialties. Popular subspecialties include, but are not limited to, pediatric hematology and oncology, which involves the care of young cancer patients; pediatric cardiology, which concentrates on the care of young people with heart defects; or pediatric psychiatry, which focuses on child-specific mental health issues.

How Do You Become a Pediatrician?

Education

It takes extensive education and training to become a pediatrician. Aspiring pediatricians train and study for eleven years or more beyond high school. After graduating from high school, candidates must earn a bachelor's degree, which usually takes four years. Then they attend medical school for four years. After successfully completing medical school, they participate in a pediatric residency program for three years. In this capacity, they work with pediatric patients in a hospital under the supervision of an experienced pediatrician. Upon completing the pediatric residency program and passing a licensing exam, they can work as general pediatricians. Individuals wanting to focus on a pediatric subspecialty must complete a second residency program in that subspecialty, which takes an additional one to three years.

To prepare for a career as a pediatrician, high school students should take classes in biology, chemistry, health, and anatomy (if available). Since pediatricians work with a diverse population, studying a foreign language is also a plus, especially one that is commonly spoken in the geographic area where the individual wants to work. In college, future pediatricians can major in any subject. Medical schools do not require that students have a particular college major. However, a premed program or a science-related major offers students a good foundation for medical school.

Admission to medical school is very competitive. There are two types of medical schools. One offers graduates a doctor of medicine degree. The other offers graduates a doctor of osteopathy degree. Graduates of either type of school can go on to be pediatricians.

Medical school requires commitment. It is expensive, and the work is challenging. During the first two years, students learn in a classroom setting. They take a wide range of life science courses, including but not limited to biology, immunology, biochemistry, anatomy, pathology, and pharmacology. Instruction in the last two years takes place in a hospital, where students observe and assist in a variety of medical specialties under the supervision of experienced physicians.

After successfully completing medical school, prospective pediatricians must complete a three-year residency program in a hospital or clinic. First-year residents are also known as interns, which signifies that they are the most junior members of a residency program. Residents work about eighty hours per week and receive a minimal salary to help cover their expenses.

Certification and Licensing

Pediatricians must be licensed. To become licensed, individuals must graduate from an accredited medical school, successfully complete a residency program, and pass either the United States Medical Licensing Examination or the Comprehensive Osteopathic Medical Licensing Examination, depending on the type of program from which they graduated. Pediatricians can also obtain

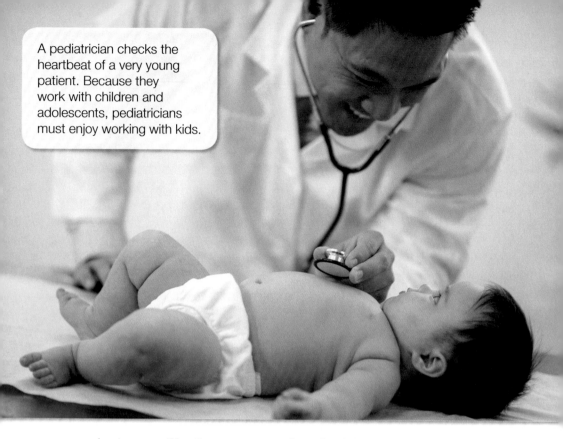

A pediatrician checks the heartbeat of a very young patient. Because they work with children and adolescents, pediatricians must enjoy working with kids.

voluntary certification as general pediatricians and in subspecialty fields by successfully completing other exams. Although not required, certification indicates that a pediatrician is an expert in the field, which helps individuals advance in their careers.

Volunteer Work and Internships

Individuals interested in becoming a pediatrician can learn about the profession and experience what it is like to work with children in a number of ways. Working or volunteering in a school, summer camp, or youth group lets individuals see whether they are comfortable working with kids. For example, Justin Smith worked with a church youth group. He recalls, "What happened during that time is that I grew to really love kids. I developed skills interacting with them that I would've otherwise never had. . . . I was still pre-med and convinced that medicine was right for me, so it seemed pretty natural that pediatrics was the way to go."

Volunteering in a hospital or children's health clinic is another valuable experience. It gives prospective pediatricians experience working with ailing children and their families and lets them see what it is like to work in a medical setting.

Skills and Personality

Pediatricians should like people, especially children. They deal with crying babies, frightened and sick children, and worried parents on a daily basis. Being patient, personable, even-tempered, and caring helps physicians calm young patients and their parents and provide them with emotional support.

Similarly, remaining cool under pressure and having a sense of humor helps pediatricians balance the ups and downs of their profession. Having a sense of humor has other advantages, too. Pediatricians often do whatever it takes to win their patients' trust and cooperation. It is not uncommon for these physicians to wear funny hats, make goofy voices, and sing silly songs to entertain and calm their patients. As Kentucky pediatrician Charles Ison explains on the Lexington Family website, "There is nothing easy about keeping kids healthy, but I try to make it as fun as I can."

Pediatricians also need good communication skills. They interact with and convey information to their patients and their patients' parents, as well as with other health care professionals. Therefore, they must be able to communicate effectively with people of all ages. They need to be good listeners, too. To make a proper diagnosis, they must actively listen to what their patients and their patients' parents tell them about current and past health issues. Moreover, because many of their patients are too young to explain what is bothering them, in order to make a correct diagnosis, pediatricians need to be very observant. This helps them notice both large and small changes in a patient's condition so that they can provide correct treatment. Perseverance, knowledge about children's health and development, and good problem-solving skills also help pediatricians solve difficult diagnostic problems.

Pediatricians should also be flexible. Their patients vary widely in age and health care issues. Therefore, these physicians need to be able to switch hats quickly. And since pediatricians deal with people of diverse backgrounds and ethnicities, it is essential that they are sensitive to and tolerant of people with different cultural values.

On the Job

Employers

Pediatricians are employed by hospitals, children's health clinics, outpatient care facilities, health maintenance organizations, and medical schools. Many are self-employed, working in solo, partnership, and group practices. According to the AAP, approximately 28 percent of all pediatricians work in group practices consisting of three to ten pediatricians.

The AAP also reports that 39 percent of pediatricians work in suburbs, 29 percent work in metropolitan areas outside of inner cities, 22 percent work in inner cities, and 10 percent work in rural communities.

Working Conditions

Pediatricians work in clean, well-lit medical facilities. In order to create a fun, positive environment for young patients, most pediatricians' offices and children's health facilities tend to have colorful, cheerful decor. On average, pediatricians work fifty hours per week, although about 25 percent work part time. Those employed by hospitals may be on call in case of emergencies and may work weekends, nights, and holidays. Self-employed pediatricians set their own hours.

Pediatricians are on their feet a lot. It is not unusual for them to be spit up on, kicked, and bitten by frightened young patients. They are exposed to body fluids and infectious diseases. Wearing gloves and washing their hands frequently helps lessen their risk of contracting or spreading an infection.

Earnings

The Bureau of Labor Statistics (BLS) reports that the average salary for a pediatrician is $172,650; the lowest-paid 10 percent of pediatricians earn about $82,670, and the highest-paid 10 percent earn more than $208,000. Earnings vary, depending on the employer and the location. According to the BLS, mean wages are highest in the following states: Mississippi, $274,470; Alaska, $265,750; Wisconsin, $259,730; South Dakota, $241,930; and Montana, $234,240.

In addition to their wages, pediatricians employed by hospitals, medical schools, and other medical facilities usually receive employee benefits such as health insurance, a retirement plan, and paid sick and vacation days. Self-employed pediatricians do not receive these benefits.

Opportunities for Advancement

Pediatricians can advance in their careers in a number of ways. Being experienced, having a good professional reputation, and holding certification help self-employed pediatricians grow their practices, which usually produces increased earnings. Salaried pediatricians generally advance on the basis of their job performance and experience and by gaining certification. In addition to increased earnings, they can advance to an administrative position as the head of pediatrics in a hospital or other health care facility. Some experienced pediatricians move from clinical practice to academic careers as part of a medical school faculty. Others work in research. Some general pediatricians go on to get further training and complete a second residency in a pediatric subspecialty, which often yields increased earnings. For example, MomMD, a website that connects female physicians, reports that the median annual earnings for pediatric surgeons is $400,591.

What Is the Future Outlook for Pediatricians?

The BLS predicts that employment opportunities for pediatricians will increase by 15 percent through 2026, which is faster than average. The best employment opportunities should be in rural and low-income areas, where there is a shortage of pediatricians.

Find Out More

American Academy of Pediatrics (AAP)
345 Park Blvd.
Itasca, IL 60143
website: www.aap.org

The AAP is a professional organization of pediatricians dedicated to the health and well-being of children and adolescents. It provides lots of information about children's health and pediatrics as a profession. It also sponsors conferences, webcasts, journals, and other publications.

American Medical Association (AMA)
AMA Plaza
330 N. Wabash Ave., Suite 39300
Chicago, IL 60611
website: www.ama-assn.org

The AMA is the largest professional organization of physicians. It provides comprehensive information about medical education and various medical professions, including pediatrics.

How to Become a Pediatrician
website: www.howtobecomeapediatrician.com

This website provides a wealth of free information for people interested in becoming a pediatrician, including information about training and education, scholarships and grants, salaries, pediatric subspecialties, duties of a pediatrician, and board certification.

Medical School Headquarters
website: https://medicalschoolhq.net

This website is authored by physicians to help individuals interested in becoming a physician reach their goal. It offers medical school students' stories, podcasts, and information about preparing for medical school, medical school admissions, and different medical specialties, including pediatrics.

Phlebotomist

What Does a Phlebotomist Do?

Phlebotomists, also known as phlebotomy technicians, are health care professionals who take blood samples from patients for research, transfusions, blood donations, and most commonly, medical tests prescribed by physicians. These blood specimens are analyzed by other medical professionals. Physicians rely on blood test results to make diagnoses, assess the effectiveness of medication, and evaluate whether a patient is getting proper nutrition.

Drawing blood is most commonly accomplished through venipuncture, a medical procedure in which phlebotomists first identify a suitable vein or other blood vessel, place a tourniquet above the area, then carefully insert an appropriately sized needle attached to a specimen tube into the vein. Phlebotomists use their technical knowledge to determine the appropriate blood vessel and needle size. For example, Massachusetts phlebotomist Yvette Coward uses tiny needles to draw blood from infants. In an interview on the All Allied Health Schools website, she

At a Glance

Phlebotomist

Minimum Educational Requirements
Postsecondary nondegree training

Personal Qualities
Good hand-eye coordination, detail oriented

Certification and Licensing
Requirements vary by state and employers

Working Conditions
Indoors in diagnostic laboratories, hospitals, and other health care facilities

Salary Range
About $24,250 to $48,030

Number of Jobs
As of 2016, about 122,700

Future Job Outlook
25 percent growth, better than average

explains, "Newborns have tiny veins that move around a lot. [For them] I use a special method. . . . It requires a small needle and a steady hand." Once the correct amount of blood is drawn, phlebotomists remove the tourniquet and apply a bandage over the puncture site in order to stanch bleeding.

In addition to taking blood samples, phlebotomists are charged with other tasks. One of the most vital is clearly labeling each specimen. All blood samples look the same. Mislabeling a sample could have serious consequences. And since the accuracy of a blood test depends on the quality of the sample, phlebotomists must also ensure that each specimen is stored properly.

Phlebotomists are also responsible for entering a record of each procedure and each patient's information into a database. In addition, they must assemble and maintain their medical instruments, keep their workstation and instruments clean and sterile, and properly dispose of used needles and other biomedical waste. Plus, because many people fear needles, an important part of a phlebotomist's job is comforting and reassuring anxious patients so that they are less nervous. As a phlebotomist explained in an interview on Just Jobs Academy, a website that provides information about different careers, "It moves me and excites me when a frightened patient . . . comes to me with great trepidation, and I am able to ease their fears, and successfully draw their blood and they exclaim 'Wow you are good! I didn't even feel it.'"

How Do You Become a Phlebotomist?

Education

Becoming a phlebotomist does not require extensive postsecondary training. High school graduates can enter this field by successfully completing a phlebotomy program at a community college, technical school, or hospital. Programs usually take just a few months to complete. To prepare for this career, high school students should take classes in health and biology. Classes in speech are also helpful, since phlebotomists need to be able to communicate effectively with their patients. A computer class is useful, too. Phlebotomists are required to have a basic understanding of how to use a computer and enter information into a database. Phlebotomy programs further require that students be at least eighteen years old.

Basic phlebotomy program course work includes classroom instruction in human anatomy and physiology, with the primary focus on the circulatory system. Instruction is also provided in blood composition, venipuncture techniques, sample labeling procedures, and medical terminology. In addition, students receive about one hundred hours of clinical training in a hospital or clinic under the supervision of a trained professional. As Texas phlebotomist Ashley Black explains in an interview on BloodTaker, a website that provides information about this career field, "I did a 9 week phlebotomy course in Bradenton, FL when I lived there. I got experience by doing morning rounds on in house patients at the hospital where the phlebotomy class was held. 4 weeks of book work and 5 weeks of learning to stick properly. During those 5 weeks I was with a mentor showing me the ropes and how to draw blood, and how to treat the patient."

Students also receive hands-on training in selecting, using, and organizing phlebotomy equipment such as different-sized needles, tourniquets, and collection tubes. They also learn about and practice safety and sanitation procedures that are necessary to keep patients and blood samples safe.

Certification and Licensing

Certification requirements for phlebotomists vary by state. As of 2018, California, Louisiana, Nevada, and Washington require that phlebotomists be certified. Many employers in other states prefer to hire certified phlebotomists. Certification indicates that a phlebotomist has demonstrated mastery of the profession. To gain certification, candidates must successfully complete a phlebotomy program and pass an exam that includes a written component and a practical component in which candidates are required to draw blood. Certification is available through a number of organizations, including but not limited to the American Society for Clinical Pathology, the National Phlebotomy Association, and the American Society of Phlebotomy Technicians.

Many phlebotomy programs expect applicants to have cardiopulmonary resuscitation (CPR) certification before entering the program. CPR certification training is offered by the Red Cross, hospitals, fire departments, and other organizations and takes about three hours to complete.

Volunteer Work and Internships

The American Red Cross and many community blood banks actively seek volunteers to assist in blood drives and in central and mobile blood banks. Doing so is a good way for aspiring phlebotomists to learn more about what phlebotomists do. Volunteering or working part time in a diagnostic laboratory, hospital, and/or health clinic are other great ways to explore this profession, as is following a phlebotomist through a typical workday.

Skills and Personality

Phlebotomists need to have excellent eye-hand coordination, steady hands, good near vision, and good manual dexterity. These traits help them perform a venipuncture successfully on the first attempt and use their equipment efficiently. Since many patients are afraid of needles and fear having blood drawn, phlebotomists should be able to work quickly in order to not prolong the patient's anxiety. Being personable helps them distract fearful patients and gain their trust. Gentleness is also vital. Many patients have sensitive skin, and handling a patient roughly can cause them pain.

Phlebotomists work in a fast-paced environment. It is not unusual for a phlebotomist to see a new patient every ten minutes, which can be exhausting. They may be on their feet for long periods. To do their job effectively, they need to be physically fit and have good stamina. And even though they may handle more than fifty cases in a day, they are expected to be compassionate and treat each patient as an individual. "There's a body attached to that arm," Lisa Scott, a Baltimore phlebotomist, jokingly explains in an article on *U.S. News & World Report*'s website.

Being detail oriented is another vital characteristic of successful phlebotomists. Phlebotomists must draw the correct amount of blood for the tests ordered, label and store each specimen correctly, and properly enter the patient's information into a database. Without careful attention to detail, blood samples might be mislabeled or misplaced, possibly causing harm to the patient. Moreover, to keep from hurting patients unnecessarily, phlebotomists must pay careful attention to detail when performing a venipuncture.

The ability to communicate effectively with patients and with other health care professionals is important, too. So are discretion and the ability to maintain privacy regarding patient medical information.

On the Job

Employers

According to the Bureau of Labor Statistics (BLS), 37 percent of phlebotomists are employed by hospitals, and 32 percent are employed by medical and diagnostic laboratories. Others are employed by blood banks, public health clinics, physicians' offices, home health care agencies, and outpatient care centers. Phlebotomists are also employed by hospices, prisons, pharmaceutical labs, and research facilities.

Working Conditions

Most phlebotomists work full time, although part-time work is available. Most work in a clean, well-lit laboratory or other medical facility. Some phlebotomists, known as mobile phlebotomists, spend a lot of time in their cars commuting. These individuals go to patients' homes to draw blood samples, which they transport to medical facilities for analysis. Those who work in hospitals and other round-the-clock health care facilities often work in eight- to twelve-hour rotating shifts. They may work three or four days per week, including weekends, holidays, and nights. Other phlebotomists work a standard five-day, forty-hour workweek.

Phlebotomists are exposed to blood-borne diseases, as well as hazardous biological waste. Also, they are at risk of needle sticks. To avoid contamination and injuries, they wear gloves, face masks, scrubs and/or lab coats, and protective eyewear; wash their hands frequently; and follow strict safety protocols. Moreover, since phlebotomists may be on their feet a good part of the day and have to bend while drawing blood, they are at risk of back and neck strains. But despite these potential risks, in a survey of phlebotomists conducted by OwlGuru.com, 72 percent of the respondents said they were satisfied with their jobs.

Earnings

According to the BLS, the lowest-paid 10 percent of phlebotomists earn less than $24,250, while the highest-paid 10 percent earn more than $48,030. It reports a median annual pay of $33,670. Earnings vary by location, employer, and a phlebotomist's experience and credentials. The BLS reports average annual wages are highest in the following states: California, $43,380; Alaska, $43,209; New Hampshire, $40,390; and Connecticut, $40,370. The American Association of Medical Personnel reports that certified phlebotomists earn 10 percent more than noncertified phlebotomists. In addition to their base salary, most phlebotomists receive employee benefits such as health insurance, a retirement plan, and paid sick and vacation days.

Opportunities for Advancement

With experience and certification, phlebotomists can advance to a supervisory position in which they oversee other phlebotomists. They can also become an instructor in a phlebotomy training program.

Some phlebotomists use their experience and knowledge of physiology, anatomy, and medical safety procedures as a stepping stone to other, more lucrative health care careers. With additional education, some become registered nurses or medical laboratory technicians who analyze blood and other bodily fluids.

What Is the Future Outlook for Phlebotomists?

The BLS predicts that employment opportunities for phlebotomists will increase by 25 percent through 2026, which is much faster than the predicted average for all employment during this period. Job prospects are expected to be greatest for certified individuals. Employment opportunities should be available throughout the United States, as well as abroad. As a phlebotomy student explains on the Texas Healthtech Institute website, "The reason I chose phlebotomy was because it's an interesting field to get into, no matter where you go in life someone is going to need their blood drawn so there will always be jobs for you to fill."

Find Out More

Center for Phlebotomy Education
PO Box 5
Corydon, IN 47112
website: www.phlebotomy.com

The Center for Phlebotomy Education is an organization that educates health care professionals and the public on all aspects of blood collecting and testing. It provides information about what phlebotomists do, phlebotomy programs and training, and certification.

National Phlebotomy Association (NPA)
1901 Brightseat Rd.
Landover, MD 20785
website: www.nationalphlebotomy.org

The NPA is concerned with educating and certifying phlebotomists. It administers a certifying test, provides online practice tests, sponsors an annual conference, and offers information about training programs.

Phlebotomist Training Center
website: www.phlebotomisttrainingcenter.com

This website serves as a resource for phlebotomists and individuals interested in becoming phlebotomists. It offers a directory of phlebotomy training programs throughout the United States, information about certification, job listings, and tips on getting hired.

Phlebotomy Careers
website: www.phlebotomycareers.net

This website is dedicated to providing information about phlebotomy careers. It has information about what phlebotomists do, what it is like to perform a venipuncture, phlebotomy training programs, certification, and salaries.

Physician Assistant

What Does a Physician Assistant Do?

A physician assistant, or PA, is a health care professional who practices medicine under the guidance of and in collaboration with a physician. Most PAs see and treat patients without a physician being present in the room, but by law, they cannot set up their own independent practices. Instead, they report to a cooperating physician, who provides them with advice and support as needed. In an interview with the editors of the book *Hot Health Care Careers,* Kara D. Larson, a PA, explains:

The M.D. is there to help when I need it for a difficult patient scenario, but I am not required to have his approval for my [treatment] plan or to have him sign my chart or prescriptions. I may go through the entire day without needing consultation or may have several complicated patients requiring his assistance. In these cases we always work as a team, making the best decisions together.

At a Glance

Physician Assistant

Minimum Educational Requirements
Master's degree

Personal Qualities
Compassionate, good problem-solving skills

Certification and Licensing
Physician assistant license

Working Conditions
Indoors, in a health care facility

Salary Range
About $66,590 to $146,260

Number of Jobs
As of 2017, about 109,220

Future Job Outlook
37 percent growth, better than average

PAs perform many of the same duties as a physician but usually handle less complex cases. Their presence makes it possible for medical practices and health care facilities to treat more patients. Although a PA's specific duties depend on the employer, state laws, and the PA's experience level, most PA duties include taking and reviewing patients' medical histories, administering medical exams, and diagnosing and treating patients. PAs also administer injections, set broken bones, stitch up wounds, and prescribe medication. They order and interpret diagnostic tests, assist in surgeries, and make rounds in hospitals. And they often counsel patients and their families about medical issues. In an interview on JobShadow.com, PA Tess Messer talks about her work as a physician assistant in an urgent care and emergency care setting. She says she sees patients "that have injuries such as burns, cuts, sprains and broken bones or illnesses such as urinary tract infections, viral infections or upper respiratory problems. . . . I may also see patients with abdominal pain, migraine headaches, threatened miscarriages or chest pain."

About half of all PAs work in primary care practices. But they are not limited to any one medical specialty field. PAs work in emergency medicine, surgery, pediatrics, oncology, and dermatology, among other fields. They are trained in a broad range of medical specialties, which gives them the flexibility to practice and switch among specialties as their interests change. For example, Russ, a Texas PA employed by the US Department of Veterans Affairs, started his career working in primary care. "Since then," he explains in an article on the department's website, "I've spent five years in psychiatry, six years in sleep research, and nine years in nuclear medicine." (Nuclear medicine is a medical specialty field that uses radioactive material to diagnose and treat certain diseases.)

How Do You Become a Physician Assistant?

Education

It takes about six years of training beyond high school to become a PA. This translates to four years of undergraduate studies, lead-

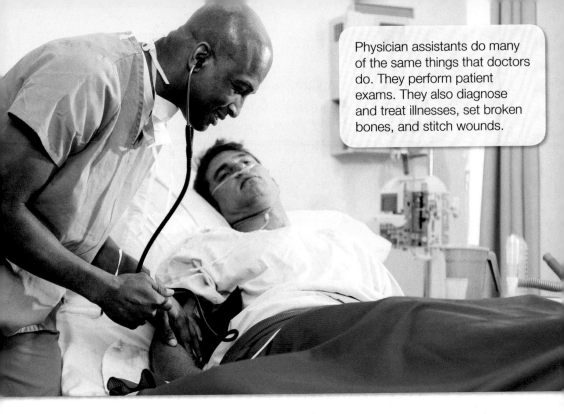

Physician assistants do many of the same things that doctors do. They perform patient exams. They also diagnose and treat illnesses, set broken bones, and stitch wounds.

ing to a bachelor's degree, followed by about twenty-six months of study in an accredited PA program, leading to a master's degree.

PA programs require candidates to have a strong background in science. Students can begin preparing for this career in high school by taking as many science classes as possible. Since PAs must be able to communicate clearly and effectively with their patients and supervising physician, speech and language arts classes are useful, too. Studying a foreign language is also a plus, especially one that is commonly spoken in the geographic area where the individual wants to work.

Admission to an accredited PA program is very competitive. Individuals can enter a PA program with any college major; however, undergraduate course work in microbiology, physiology, anatomy, and chemistry, among other sciences, are common prerequisites for admission. Therefore, many applicants major in biology or another life science to meet admission requirements. In addition, most programs require applicants to have previous work or volunteer experience in health care.

PA programs mix classroom and laboratory instruction with clinical experience. The first year of study usually consists of lectures and labs in subjects such as anatomy, medical ethics, pathology, and pharmacology, among others. For the remainder of their training, students get practical experience working with patients under the supervision of a physician in a variety of medical specialties. In many cases, students take this clinical training along with medical school interns.

Certification and Licensing

All states require PAs to be licensed. To become licensed, candidates must successfully complete an accredited PA program and pass the Physician Assistant National Certifying Exam. It tests a candidate's medical knowledge and clinical skills. Those who pass the exam are awarded the title Physician Assistant–Certified (PA-C), which allows them to practice medicine under the supervision of a physician.

Volunteer Work and Internships

Individuals interested in a career as a PA are encouraged to volunteer or work in a hospital, physician's office, or other health care facility. Doing so gives individuals the opportunity to explore the medical field, observe and interact with PAs, and gain the type of health care experience that is required for admission to most PA programs. Other activities, like volunteering at a blood drive or a disaster relief event, riding along with local emergency medical technicians, or working with special-needs children and adults, also help fulfill admission requirements. In addition, many PA programs require or prefer that candidates have spent time shadowing, or following, a PA-C. This is a good way for individuals to learn exactly what PAs do and explore the variety of medical specialties open to them. As Larson advises, "Shadow multiple PAs in various specialties and settings to understand how PAs function. . . . If possible, work as a medical assistant or a patient care technician in a hospital. This is not the most glamorous job (it involves bed changes and patient baths) but it will give you a glimpse into the health care setting as well as teach you basic skills."

Skills and Personality

PAs should be able to work independently and as part of a team. In order to make a correct diagnosis and administer appropriate treatment, they must trust their own technical skill, have good problem-solving abilities, and be decisive. At the same time, they should be perceptive enough to know when they need assistance and feel comfortable asking for and following the advice and instructions of their supervising physician.

Being personable, considerate, and compassionate are also vital. These traits help PAs calm distraught patients and win their trust, which makes it easier to treat them. Good listening and communication skills are useful, too. In order to make an accurate diagnosis, PAs must listen carefully when patients describe their symptoms. And they should be able to explain diagnoses and treatments to patients and share information with physicians and other health care professionals. In an interview on the Muse, a job and career website, New York PA Nicole LaCoste explains, "You're constantly interacting with colleagues and patients every day. You have to be able to describe medical terms in layman's terms, and you must be confident and comfortable talking about awkward or uncomfortable things in a way that makes patients trust you, and open up to you. Part of that is having a personable persona and being relatable."

On the Job

Employers

PAs are employed throughout the United States. According to the Bureau of Labor Statistics (BLS), approximately 60 percent of all PAs are employed in physicians' offices, and about 25 percent are employed by hospitals. PAs are also employed by outpatient care facilities, public health clinics, home health care agencies, prisons, government agencies, the military, and educational institutions.

Working Conditions

PAs usually work in clean, well-lit health care facilities. Many work a five-day, forty-hour week, which may include evenings and weekends, depending on the employer. Opportunities to work part time are also available. PAs who work in hospitals or other round-the-clock health care facilities often work in eight- to twelve-hour rotating shifts. They may work three or four days per week, including nights, holidays, and weekends, and they may be on call at other times. For instance, a PA who works in a large urgent care facility reports that she works twelve-hour shifts with two days on and two days off.

PAs face some health risks as part of their job. They are in direct contact with sick and injured patients, and they handle needles. Exposure to harmful pathogens, infected bodily fluids, and needle sticks is part of the job. To ward off infection, they wear protective clothing, gloves, and face masks and wash their hands frequently. To protect themselves from needle sticks, they follow strict guidelines in handling needles.

Earnings

According to the BLS, the lowest-paid 10 percent of PAs earn less than $66,590, while the highest-paid 10 percent earn more than $146,260. The BLS reports the median salary to be $104,860. Wages vary, depending on the employer, the location of the job, and the PA's experience. Average wages are highest in the following states: Washington, $120,200; New Jersey, $119,260; Nevada, $119,210; North Dakota, $117,500; and Hawaii, $116,660. Wages tend to be higher in metropolitan areas than in rural areas.

PAs usually receive employee benefits such as health and dental insurance, paid sick and vacation days, and a retirement plan. Some employers offer a monetary sign-on bonus for new hires and student loan repayment assistance.

Opportunities for Advancement

As their experience and clinical skills grow, PAs can expect to be given pay raises and greater autonomy and responsibilities. Some advance to administrative positions in hospitals and other large health care facilities. Some become instructors in PA training programs. Others continue their education and become licensed physicians. PAs can also make lateral changes in their careers by switching between specialty fields as their interests change. Such changes often come with a pay raise, improved working conditions, and/or a more flexible work schedule.

What Is the Future Outlook for Physician Assistants?

This is a rapidly growing career field. According to the BLS, employment opportunities for PAs is predicted to increase by 37 percent through 2026, which is much faster than the predicted average for all employment during this period. With a growing and aging population, the demand for health care services is expected to increase. Currently, shortages of physicians exist in primary care practices and across other specialty fields in some areas of the country. Since PAs can provide many of the same services as physicians and can be trained in a shorter period of time, they are expected to play a growing role in providing medical services in the future. Opportunities should be greatest in primary care practices and in inner cities and rural areas. In an article on the *Forbes* website, Jim Stone, the president of Medicus, a national medical staffing and placement firm, explains, "As competition intensifies for primary care physicians, we may start to see more hospitals and health systems back-filling primary care physician openings with PAs . . . rather than going understaffed in primary care for an extended period of time. It's already happening . . . and may become a more common occurrence in the future."

Find Out More

American Academy of Physician Assistants (AAPA)
950 N. Washington St.
Alexandria, VA 22314
e-mail: aapa@aapa.org
website: www.aapa.org

The AAPA is a professional organization made up of PAs and PA students. It offers lots of information about PA education programs, certification, and this career field.

National Commission on Certification of Physician Assistants (NCCPA)
12000 Findley Rd., Suite 100
Johns Creek, GA 30097
e-mail: nccpa@nccpa.net
website: www.nccpa.net

The NCCPA is the organization that administers the PA certifying exam and awards certification. It offers information about what PAs do and the certifying exam, as well as providing job postings.

PA Journey
website: www.pajourney.com

PA Journey is a blog authored by a PA student. It provides a wide range of information about getting admitted to a PA education program, PA student experiences, preparing for certification exams, finding a job, and what it is like to be a PA.

Physician Assistant Education Association (PAEA)
655 K St. NW, Suite 700
Washington, DC 20001
e-mail: info@PAEAonline.org
website: www.paeaonline.org

The PAEA is a national organization representing PA education programs. It offers information about a career as a PA; training programs; financial aid, scholarships, and grants; certification and practice certification exam materials; and publications, forums, and workshops.

Interview with a Massage Therapist

Kim Carlsen is a self-employed massage therapist in Las Cruces, New Mexico. She has worked as a massage therapist for more than twenty years. She spoke with the author about her career.

Q: Why did you become a massage therapist?
A: The health care field has always interested me. I became a massage therapist because the idea of being able to work with the public, work with people, help with their health issues, help with relaxation; that really appealed to me. I also liked the fact that I could set my own schedule since I had a baby at the time. So, I could work around being with him more and that was nice.

Q: Can you describe a typical workday?
A: First off, I check to see how many appointments I have that day. If any clients need anything special, I prepare that. I get my table ready with clean sheets, pillows. I make sure I have my massage cream containers filled, clean the massage area, the waiting room, and the bathroom—just make sure the [massage therapy] room is comfortable temperature wise. I pick out my music to play. I usually do two or three appointments a day, so I repeat that little routine making up the table for each one. When the client comes in I check in with them about any current health issues, aches and pains, that type of thing. If it's a new client, I have a health questionnaire I have them fill out. Once this is all taken care of, I help my clients onto the table and work on them.

Q: What do you like most and least about your job?

A: One of the things I like most is that I've become friends with most of my clients. Some of my clients have been with me a long time. I have clients I have been working on for seventeen or eighteen years. Another thing I like is when I get positive feedback from my clients, that I helped them. I also like the flexibility of being in business for myself, which makes me able to schedule clients when it is convenient for me.

What I like least is a tough question, because I really like what I do. Although, sometimes a client comes a few times and then never comes back, and I wonder why, if it was something I did. Also, there are times when I don't have a lot of clients because of holidays and vacations, and then I don't make too much money because I'm self-employed. But otherwise, there is no downside.

Q: What personal qualities do you find valuable for this type of work?

A: A big one is you have to enjoy being close to people. You have to not mind touching bodies of all shapes and sizes. You have to be very aware of body mechanics so you don't injure your client or yourself, and you have to be able to relate to people one on one.

Q: What advice do you have for students who might be interested in this career?

A: They should get massages from several different people to see what different massages and techniques are like. Massage therapists have to be licensed [in most states] and there's a national certificate, so they should absolutely go to massage therapy school. I think it is helpful when you are first starting out to work in an established massage studio with other established therapists, to learn from them, and to get walk-in clients that will come into an established studio, like overflow clients and walk-ins, which helps you to establish your own client base before striking out on your own. And, no matter whether you work for yourself or for someone else just make sure the massage area is warm, welcoming, and calming for your clients.

Q: How did you train for your career?
A: I did go to massage therapy school. It was 750 hours. I think it was nine months long. While I was training I practiced by working on a lot of family and friends. My training didn't end when I finished school. Every state is different, but I have to have sixteen hours of continuing education every two years to maintain my license, and I have to have liability insurance.

Q: Do you have anything else to add?
A: It takes a while to build a clientele and get established, so don't get discouraged. There are lots of classes to help beginning therapists with marketing. New therapists should take advantage of professional organizations. They offer a lot of good business advice and continuing education opportunities.

Other Jobs in Health Care

Anesthesiologist
Art therapist
Athletic trainer
Audiologist
Biomedical engineer
Biomedical equipment
  technician
Chiropractor
Cytotechnologist
Dentist
Dietitian
Emergency medical
  technician
Exercise physiologist
Genetics counselor
Health educator
Home health aide
Licensed practical nurse
Medical coder
Mental health counselor
Music therapist
Naturopathic physician

Nuclear medicine technologist
Nurse's aide
Ophthalmic medical technician
Optician
Optometrist
Oral and maxillofacial surgeon
Orthodontist
Pathologist
Perfusionist
Pharmacist
Pharmacy technician
Physical therapist
Physical therapist assistant
Physician
Podiatrist
Radiologic technician
Registered nurse
Rehabilitation counselor
Respiratory therapist
Social worker
Speech-language pathologist
Veterinarian

Editor's Note: The US Department of Labor's Bureau of Labor Statistics provides information about hundreds of occupations. The agency's *Occupational Outlook Handbook* describes what these jobs entail, the work environment, education and skill requirements, pay, future outlook, and more. The *Occupational Outlook Handbook* may be accessed online at www.bls.gov/ooh.

Index